CONFRONTING HEREDITARY BREAST AND OVARIAN CANCER

A JOHNS HOPKINS PRESS HEALTH BOOK

CONFRONTING HEREDITARY BREAST AND OVARIAN CANCER

Identify Your Risk, Understand Your Options, Change Your Destiny

SUE FRIEDMAN, D.V.M.

REBECCA SUTPHEN, M.D.

KATHY STELIGO

Foreword by Mark H. Greene, M.D.

ENDORSED BY
FACING OUR RISK OF CANCER EMPOWERED
(FORCE)

THE JOHNS HOPKINS UNIVERSITY PRESS
Baltimore

616.994
Fri

© 2012 The Johns Hopkins University Press
All rights reserved. Published 2012
Printed in the United States of America on acid-free paper
9 8 7 6 5 4 3 2 1

The Johns Hopkins University Press
2715 North Charles Street
Baltimore, Maryland 21218-4363
www.press.jhu.edu

A catalog record for this book is available from the British Library.

Special discounts are available for bulk purchases of this book. For more information, please contact Special Sales at 410-516-6936 or specialsales@press.jhu.edu.

The Johns Hopkins University Press uses environmentally friendly book materials, including recycled text paper that is composed of at least 30 percent post-consumer waste, whenever possible.

LIBRARY OF CONGRESS CATALOGING-IN-PUBLICATION DATA

Friedman, Sue.
  Confronting hereditary breast and ovarian cancer : identify your risk, understand your options, change your destiny / Sue Friedman, Rebecca Sutphen, and Kathy Steligo ; foreword by Mark H. Greene.
    p.   cm. — (A Johns Hopkins Press health book)
  Includes bibliographical references and index.
  ISBN-13: 978-1-4214-0407-3 (hardcover : alk. paper)
  ISBN-13: 978-1-4214-0408-0 (pbk. : alk. paper)
  ISBN-10: 1-4214-0407-9 (hardcover : alk. paper)
  ISBN-10: 1-4214-0408-7 (pbk. : alk. paper)
  1. Breast—Cancer—Genetic aspects—Popular works. 2. Breast—Cancer—Risk factors—Popular works. 3. Breast—Cancer—Prevention—Popular works. 4. Ovaries—Cancer—Genetic aspects—Popular works. 5. Ovaries—Cancer—Risk factors—Popular works. 6. Ovaries—Cancer—Prevention—Popular works. I. Sutphen, Rebecca. II. Steligo, Kathy. III. Title.
  RC280.B8F739 2012
  616.99'449042—dc23   2011019918

4|8|13

Contents

Foreword

IT IS BOTH FITTING and instructive that *Confronting Hereditary Breast and Ovarian Cancer* should come to us now, some seventeen years after the identification of the BRCA1 and BRCA2 cancer-susceptibility genes: fitting in that it meets an urgent need for a trusted source of authoritative information, and instructive in demonstrating how far the hereditary breast and ovarian cancer (HBOC) field has progressed since those paradigm-altering observations were made. This important guide can direct our research focus in the years ahead, as we strive to optimize quality of life, management, and survival among persons at increased genetic risk of breast and ovarian cancer.

A glance at the table of contents reveals a comprehensive list of the challenges faced by all carriers of rare cancer-susceptibility genes, ranging from an introduction to genetic principles, through risk assessment and genetic testing, to surgical and medical management, with each topic beautifully illustrated using the specific example of HBOC. The substance of each chapter is impeccably accurate, and the authors honestly acknowledge the limits of our current understanding of this incredibly complex disorder. Where all the facts are not yet known, they present the carefully considered best medical judgment of investigators and providers who have devoted their careers to the study of HBOC, informed and shaped by those carrying BRCA mutations as well as the important people in their lives.

The voices of these women are heard loud and clear throughout the text; they give the information presented here a genuine and legitimate quality that will surely resonate with readers as they struggle to come to terms with what it means to carry a BRCA1/2 mutation. Consequently, the tone of the book is an extraordinary combination of indisputably authoritative and insightful information, presented in a voice that is calm, clear, direct, balanced, realistic, and yet optimistic. Readers will know that, without a doubt, they are hearing from people who have been there and survived, people who now share their hard-won wisdom and insight in an effort to ease the path for those who follow in their footsteps.

The authors employ several novel organizational strategies in an effort to convey their message as clearly as possible. "Expert View" sections give voice to leaders in HBOC research and care; "My Story" sections share the heartfelt words of women who have direct experience with the topic under discussion; and "The FORCE Perspective" sections describe the current positions of the organization that has led the effort to give women from HBOC families a voice in their own fate. All three add greatly to the effectiveness of the educational effort embodied by this book. It is filled with pearls of wisdom that can only come from those who speak from firsthand experience. Examples include the unassailable assertion that genetic counseling must be seen as an ongoing, open-ended process rather than a one-time event, and the discussion of the pros and cons of various surgical approaches to risk-reducing mastectomy.

As a clinician and investigator who has been involved in evaluating HBOC families for the past thirty-five years, since long before the identification of BRCA1/2, I remember all too well the frustrations we faced due to the lack of data upon which to base management recommendations for the pioneering women who participated in our research studies in the 1970s and 1980s. I also remember the anguish of women from multiple-case families who *all* regarded themselves as destined to develop breast and/or ovarian cancer, because of our inability to identify the specific family members who were at genetic risk. It was heartbreaking to realize that many of the women from that era who elected risk-reducing breast and ovarian surgery likely did *not* carry the mutated gene that formed the basis for their family's cancer risk. Perhaps the single greatest difficulty faced by BRCA mutation carriers as they struggled to manage their risk was the lack of reliable, consistent, authoritative information from their healthcare providers, with contradictory recommendations being distressingly common.

This book should go a long way toward making that unacceptable status quo a thing of the past. And for that, future generations of BRCA mutation carriers can thank the indomitable and tireless FORCE organization for insisting that women have the information they need to maximize their long-term survival.

MARK H. GREENE, M.D.
CHIEF, CLINICAL GENETICS BRANCH
NATIONAL CANCER INSTITUTE
BETHESDA, MARYLAND

Acknowledgments

THE AUTHORS gratefully acknowledge the input, support, and enthusiasm of the many people who helped make this book possible. Thank you to all who shared stories and to each and every one of the healthcare professionals and researchers who took the time to contribute an "Expert View."

We appreciate permission to use the filmmaker's statement and a quotation from Kartemquin Films' *In the Family*.

A special thanks to those who read and improved what we wrote, including Diljeet Singh, M.D., Susan Domchek, M.D., Minas Chrysopoulo, M.D., Wendy Rubinstein, M.D., Ph.D., Monica Alvarado, M.S., C.G.C., Jana Pruski-Clark, M.S., C.G.C., Rachel Nussbaum, M.S., C.G.C., Tiffani DeMarco, M.S., Sally Scroggs, R.D., L.D., Jennifer Leib, Sc.M., C.G.C., David Winchester, M.D., Amy Fort, Rose Kovatch, Dan Maysey, Barbara Pfeiffer, and Robin Pugh Yi. Ginger Gardner, M.D., graciously provided timely reviews to help us meet deadlines.

And finally, we are indebted to the extraordinary support of Allison Kurian, M.D., Tim Rebbeck, Ph.D., and Victoria Seewaldt, M.D.

Introduction

THESE DAYS, IT'S NOT UNCOMMON for more than one person in a family to have cancer. Most cancers are not hereditary, but if you or your relatives have been diagnosed, you might wonder how you can learn if the cancers are random or due to some inherited predisposition. Should you be tested to determine whether you've inherited changes in the BReast CAncer1 and BReast CAncer2 (BRCA1 and BRCA2) genes you've heard so much about? Are other risk factors at play? If a test reveals that you have a greater-than-average cancer risk, what should you do to remain cancer free? If you're facing treatment for a diagnosis, how would knowledge of an inherited risk affect you during treatment and beyond?

Sorting through scientific terms, understanding risk management, and dealing with the emotions of it all can be overwhelming. Still, you deserve a "normal" life that isn't disrupted by fears about cancer. If you've inherited high risk or been diagnosed with hereditary breast or ovarian cancer, you face difficult decisions about what is best for you now and in the long term, and you need credible information to make them. You're not the first person to have these concerns or ask these questions. As cancer survivors and women who have pursued genetic counseling and testing, we've asked these same questions ourselves. And as professionals who deal with these medical issues daily, we help people who struggle with the same concerns. We know that confronting hereditary cancer can be a complex, confusing, and highly individual journey. We also know that you can take actions to gain control of your health.

Facing Our Risk of Cancer Empowered (FORCE) was founded on the principle that no one should face hereditary cancer alone. Since 1999, the nonprofit organization has been a trusted source of information, support, and resources for individuals and families affected by hereditary breast and ovarian cancers. For just as long, people have been asking when we would compile that knowledge and expertise into a book. Now we have—you're holding it.

As we put fingers to keyboards, we considered how to develop the most comprehensive and objective resource possible for people wondering what to do about their high cancer risk. We began with our existing base of information, to which we added relevant input from the world's leading cancer and genetics experts. As we wrote about practical risk-reducing alternatives, our goal was to dispel myths and misinformation about hereditary cancer. Then we added a few meaningful extras: personal stories from individuals who have dealt with these same issues and confronted the same agonizing decisions you now face, clarification about insurance coverage and discrimination, unique insights we've learned from serving our community, and a summary of each chapter's key points. The result is *Confronting Hereditary Breast and Ovarian Cancer,* our up-to-date composite of research, insight, and inspiration, all bundled together to provide answers, whether you're new to the subject or well versed.

Decisions about hereditary cancer may be the most difficult you'll ever make. But you needn't make them alone. This book is your road map through the maze of alternatives that comes with living in a high-risk body. We suggest you start at the beginning and read through consecutive chapters. Page by page, you'll sort through and absorb all the information you need, gaining clarity to make the best decisions you can for you and your family. We've organized the book into four main parts:

- "Understanding Cancer, Genetics, and Risk" introduces cancer, specifically breast and ovarian cancer, inherited and acquired genetic damage, and hereditary cancer syndromes that run in families.
- "Assessing Your Risk" explores the value of genetic counseling and genetic testing to determine whether you or someone in your family has a BRCA mutation. This section describes what you can expect from

genetic counseling and testing, which family members should be tested first, how to interpret test results, and how to decipher your range of risk.

- "Managing Your Risk" helps you understand and assess your options for managing and lowering your cancer risk and choose alternatives that are right for you. It also provides decision-making tools and compares different strategies for reducing risk.
- "Living with BRCA" identifies strategies for dealing with the day-to-day and long-term emotional and physical issues of cancer survivors and high-risk individuals. You'll find suggestions for discussing your BRCA status and dealing with the parental guilt of potentially passing along a mutation to your children. You'll read about fertility and family planning issues, sexuality, sensuality, and dating after mastectomy or oophorectomy. Our chapter devoted to men's issues provides information about specific screening, diagnosis, and treatment.

Knowledge can be both empowering and comforting. In many cases, it is lifesaving. And although there is no single right answer for all readers—we are all individuals with our own concerns, circumstances, and priorities that affect our decisions—the information you'll find in this book will demystify the complexities of hereditary cancer.

We can't make decisions for you, but we do the next best thing: we explain all sides of the hereditary cancer story—how to know if you have exceptionally high risk, alternatives for managing that risk, and the benefits and downsides of each choice. You needn't spend hours surfing the Internet looking for information, trying to decipher studies on medical sites, defining terms and attempting to distinguish between hype and fact. We've done that for you. We don't have perfect medical solutions—no one does at this time—but we can help you potentially change your destiny by equipping you with resources, facts, and support.

Be informed. Be empowered. Be well.

SUE FRIEDMAN, D.V.M.
REBECCA SUTPHEN, M.D.
KATHY STELIGO

PART ONE UNDERSTANDING CANCER, GENETICS, AND RISK

Chapter 1 **Breast and**

Ovarian Cancer

Basics

FROM A STRICTLY SCIENTIFIC PERSPECTIVE, women have breasts to feed their babies. Yet, for most of us, our breasts are much more than milk-producing glands. Our emotional attachment to our breasts is considerable, increasing as we move from puberty to maturity. Breasts enhance our physical form, give us sexual pleasure, and help us forge a close maternal bond as we nourish our infants. Although our ovaries aren't as visible, their reproductive role is more significant, from our first menstrual cycle to monthly fertility and, finally, our change of life. A woman's breasts and ovaries are uniquely feminine and intensely personal; the threat of cancer in either is particularly scary.

Most Cancers Aren't Hereditary

People with cancer are often surprised if none of their relatives has been diagnosed, but most cancers aren't hereditary. The majority are sporadic. They develop from damage that our genes acquire (not inherit) as we age. Genes are fundamental to all living organisms, including humans. They contain instructions for critical body functions and hold all hereditary information that is passed from parent to child. Inherited genetic changes called *mutations* cause about 5 to 10 percent of breast cancers and 12 percent of ovarian cancers. Most of these hereditary breast and ovarian cancers are caused by mutations in two specific genes, BReast CAncer 1 (BRCA1) and BReast CAncer 2 (BRCA2).[1] These mutations are *familial* (they run in families). They account for only a small percentage of breast and ovarian cancers, yet their presence greatly increases a woman's risk for both. Multiple diagnoses in a family also

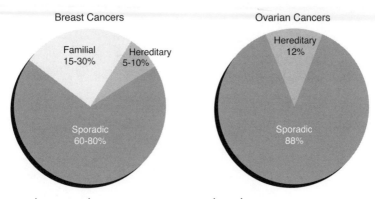

Breast Cancers   Ovarian Cancers

Breast Cancers:
Familial 15-30%
Hereditary 5-10%
Sporadic 60-80%

Ovarian Cancers:
Hereditary 12%
Sporadic 88%

Most breast and ovarian cancers aren't hereditary

raise a woman's risk. A family history of breast cancer, even when there is no BRCA mutation in the family, increases breast cancer risk. A strong history of ovarian cancer elevates a woman's risk for that disease.

Sporadic and hereditary cancers differ in important ways that may affect healthcare decisions:

- Hereditary cancer often occurs at an earlier age than the sporadic form of the same cancer.
- Recommendations for cancer screening and risk reduction can differ, and should begin at a younger age for individuals who have an inherited gene mutation or a family history of cancer.
- Multiple family members may inherit the same gene mutation that increases risk for certain hereditary cancers.
- Children can inherit a parent's gene mutation.

Throughout the remainder of this book, you'll learn how inherited mutations or a family history affect your risk for cancer and how you can manage that risk.

An Introduction to Breast Cancer

More than a million new cases of breast cancer occur each year worldwide. In the United States, it's the second most commonly diagnosed cancer (after skin cancer) among women, and it causes more

Table 1. U.S. breast cancer statistics

Lifetime risk of breast cancer	1 in 8
New cases expected in 2010	261,100*
Estimated deaths in 2010	39,840

Source: American Cancer Society, "What are the risk factors for breast cancer?" www.cancer.org/Cancer/BreastCancer/DetailedGuide/breast-cancer-risk-factors. *Includes 207,090 new cases of invasive breast cancer and 54,010 new cases of noninvasive breast cancer.

deaths than any other cancer except lung cancer. It also affects men, although far less frequently—less than 1 percent of all breast cancers occur in men.

Breast cancer deaths have declined since 1990 because of increased awareness, better methods of early detection, and advances in treatment. Yet too many women, about forty thousand every year, still die from this disease. In the 1970s, a woman living in the United States had a 1 in 11 chance of developing breast cancer in her lifetime; those odds steadily worsened over the next two decades. Since 1999, breast cancer has decreased among women over age 50, while

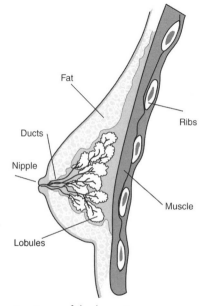

Anatomy of the breast

rates among younger women remain unchanged. Today, an average woman's lifetime risk of developing breast cancer is 1 in 8 (approximately 12.5 percent) (see table 1).

Breast cancer almost always begins in the lobules (the glands that produce milk) or the ducts (the tubes that carry milk to the nipple). Cancer usually develops over several years, typically without pain or other noticeable symptoms, until it shows up as a suspicious calcification on a mammogram or is found as a lump during a breast exam by a woman or her doctor. A tumor may show itself as it grows: a lump or area of thickness, a change in the size or shape of the breast, a skin irritation or dryness that refuses to heal, or unusual tenderness or discharge from the nipple. These same changes often occur with other conditions and don't always signal breast cancer.

Types of Breast Cancer

Tumors are either in situ, or invasive. In situ, meaning "in place," refers to early stage breast cancer that remains within the ducts or the lobules. Nearly all women diagnosed with in situ breast tumors are cured—their cancer isn't likely to return. Invasive tumors are more worrisome, because if cancerous cells reach the bloodstream or lymph nodes, they can *metastasize* (spread) to the liver, bones, lungs, and other organs. Treatment is then more involved, and remission or cure is less likely.

Ductal carcinoma in situ (DCIS) develops in the milk ducts. About 1 in 5 new breast cancers are DCIS, the earliest stage and most commonly diagnosed in situ breast cancer. Too small to be felt, DCIS is usually found by mammography or magnetic resonance imaging (MRI). Early detection is important because, left untreated, some DCIS develops into invasive breast cancer and may metastasize. If you have DCIS, your risk of developing a new breast cancer or recurrence is higher than that of someone who has never been diagnosed.

Lobular carcinoma in situ (LCIS) isn't considered a true breast cancer. Usually diagnosed in premenopausal women, LCIS involves abnormal cells that signal a higher-than-average risk of developing invasive breast cancer. Rarely found by mammography, LCIS is usually discovered during a breast biopsy to explore a lump, *microcalcification* (the residue from rapidly dividing cells that may signal an early cancer), or other abnormality.

Invasive ductal carcinoma (IDC) is cancer that has spread beyond the ducts to the surrounding breast tissue. It's the most common breast cancer, accounting for about 80 percent of all cases. Although women of any age can develop IDC, it's more often found after age 55.

Invasive lobular carcinoma (ILC) begins in the lobules and spreads to the breast tissue. Only 10 percent of invasive breast cancers are ILC, which is more often diagnosed in women who are age 60 and older.

Inflammatory breast cancer (IBC) accounts for only 1 to 3 percent of breast cancers. It often begins with swelling or reddening of the breast rather than a lump. IBC can grow very quickly—symptoms may worsen in a single day—so it's very important to recognize the signs of this disease and seek prompt treatment. IBC tends to occur at an earlier age than most other breast cancers, on average at age 56 for white women and age 52 for African American women, who are more likely to develop IBC.

> ## STAGING CANCERS
>
> By defining a tumor's size, how far it has spread, and whether lymph nodes are involved, *oncologists* (cancer experts) *stage* cancers to develop a treatment plan and predict a patient's long-term outcome. Stage 0 is sometimes called pre-invasive cancer and includes DCIS. Stages 1 to 3 depend on tumor size and lymph node involvement. Stage 4 cancers have metastasized and invaded other organs.

Paget's disease spreads from the ducts to the nipple or areola and is often characterized by a dry, scaly, itchy, or red patch. It usually affects women 50 and older. Paget's is quite rare, less than 1 percent of all breast cancers. Because most women with Paget's disease also have DCIS or invasive breast cancer, early diagnosis is very important.

Tumor Characteristics

Cancers have different characteristics, and no two are exactly alike. Some are slow growing and predictable. Others grow aggressively. A tumor's size, stage, and growth pattern determine how it's treated. Some breast cancers have hormone receptors: protein molecules in the cells that bind to estrogen and progesterone and act like on-off switches for tumor growth. Cancers with hormone receptors are referred to as *estrogen receptor–positive* (ER+) or *progesterone receptor–positive* (PR+); they respond well to antihormone treatments that either reduce the amount of estrogen or progesterone in the body or block a tumor's ability to use these hormones to grow. ER+ and PR+ tumors usually occur in women who are older than age 50. They're also the most common tumors in women with BRCA2 mutations, regardless of age. Tumors without estrogen or progesterone receptors are said to be receptor-negative (ER– and PR–); they don't respond as well to antihormone therapies. Up to a third of breast cancers *overexpress* (make too much) *HER2/neu*, a protein that promotes the growth of cancer cells. Treatment includes medications that specifically target HER2 receptors.

About 15 percent of breast cancers are *triple-negative*; they're not sensitive to estrogen, progesterone, or HER2. These cancers occur more often before age 50, especially in women who are African American or who have a BRCA1 mutation. Triple-negative tumors don't respond to hormone therapies or treatments that target the HER2 protein. Research of potential new drugs to treat triple-negative breast cancers is promising.

An Introduction to Ovarian Cancer

Ovaries are two small glands that are part of the female reproductive system, along with the fallopian tubes, vagina, and uterus. During puberty, a girl's ovaries begin to produce estrogen, progesterone, and testosterone as she develops into a sexually mature woman, and

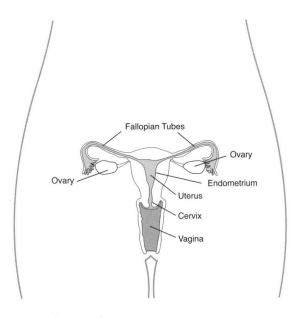

Female reproductive system

her body prepares for childbearing. During monthly ovulation, one ovary releases an egg, which then travels through the fallopian tube to the uterus. If the egg is fertilized with sperm, conception occurs. If it remains unfertilized, it dries up and is shed during menstruation.

Our ovaries produce estrogen, progesterone, and other hormones that control fertility, support pregnancy, and affect other critical body functions during our reproductive years. Ovaries keep bones strong, boost metabolism, stimulate sex drive, and regulate the menstrual cycle. As you age and reach menopause, your ovaries gradually produce fewer hormones, until your menstrual periods stop.

We don't know exactly why cancer develops in the ovaries. Some experts theorize that the monthly process of releasing eggs may cause damage that eventually leads to cancer. Others believe that the balance of progesterone compared to estrogen may play a role in protecting the ovaries from cancer. The risk for ovarian cancer increases as we age, and most ovarian cancers develop after menopause. Half develop in women over age 63.

Ovarian cancer isn't as common as breast cancer, but the ovaries are tucked away deep in the body, and without reliable early detection, tumors aren't usually discovered until they've progressed to an advanced stage and are more difficult to treat. Most early stage breast and ovarian cancers are cured, yet only about 20 percent of ovarian cancers are discovered at an early stage before they've spread to other tissue or organs. Although women diagnosed in the earliest stages have a five-year survival rate of nearly 93 percent—nearly double what it was twenty years ago—the number of ovarian cancer cases found early remains small (see table 2).

Table 2. U.S. ovarian cancer statistics

Lifetime risk of invasive ovarian cancer	1 in 70
New cases expected in 2010	21,880
Estimated deaths in 2010	13,850

Source: American Cancer Society, "What are the key statistics about ovarian cancer?" www.cancer.org/Cancer/OvarianCancer/DetailedGuide/ovarian-cancer-key-statistics.

Ovarian Cancer Symptoms

Ovarian cancer has been termed "the silent killer" because it was falsely believed to be a disease without warning signs. But research confirms that many women experience symptoms several months before they're diagnosed. Being aware of symptoms could lead to earlier diagnosis. Symptoms can include:

- bloating
- pelvic or abdominal pain
- difficulty eating or feeling full quickly
- change in urinary urgency or frequency
- fatigue
- indigestion
- back pain
- pain during intercourse
- constipation
- menstrual irregularities

These symptoms can be subtle and easily ignored or mistakenly associated with bladder or digestive conditions. Symptoms are particularly significant if they're new, occur every other day or more frequently, and last more than two weeks. If your doctor treats you for something other than ovarian cancer, and your symptoms linger or become worse, quickly get a second opinion from a gynecologic expert. Surviving ovarian cancer depends on early detection.

Ovarian and Related Cancers

About 90 percent of ovarian cancers (and most hereditary ovarian cancers) are believed to begin in the epithelial cells that form a thin layer of tissue covering the ovary. When experts refer to ovarian cancer risk, symptoms, and diagnosis, they're including *primary peritoneal* and *fallopian tube* cancers, which are treated similarly to ovarian cancer.

Fallopian tube cancer. Fallopian tube cancer affects only three hundred to four hundred women in the United States annually, usually between ages 50 and 60. Symptoms may include abdominal pain or pressure and unusual vaginal bleeding (especially after menopause) or discharge. Emerging research suggests that many hereditary ovarian cancers may actually be fallopian tube cancers that have spread to the ovaries; distinguishing between the two can be challenging. The lifetime risk for BRCA-related fallopian tube cancer is relatively low, about 6 percent.[2]

Primary peritoneal cancer. Primary peritoneal cancer begins outside the ovaries in the peritoneum, a thin membrane lining the abdomen, and can very quickly spread to other tissues. The peritoneum is made up of the same type of epithelial cells that line the ovaries, so it's not surprising that peritoneal cancer looks and behaves like ovarian cancer, has similar symptoms, and is treated as stage 3 or 4 ovarian cancer. Women with high risk for ovarian cancer, particularly those with inherited risk, are more likely to also develop peritoneal cancer, although it occurs rarely. The lifetime risk for BRCA-related primary peritoneal cancer is 2 to 6 percent.[3]

Other Hereditary Cancers

Families with BRCA1 or BRCA2 mutations have increased risk for breast and ovarian cancer. They may also have higher-than-average risk for other cancers. (Screening recommendations for these cancers are discussed in chapter 8. Other cancers caused by mutations in different genes, which can run in families, are discussed in chapter 4.)

Pancreatic Cancer

The pancreas aids digestion, secretes insulin, and regulates your body's sugar level. Because the pancreas is positioned behind the stomach, tumors are difficult to detect. Even when it's diagnosed early, this disease spreads quickly and is difficult to treat. Risk factors include:

- aging, especially after age 60
- being overweight or obese
- smoking
- diabetes
- being African American
- a family history of certain hereditary cancers
- a personal or family history of pancreatic cancer

Pancreatic cancer is uncommon; the average person's lifetime risk is just 1 percent. Family history is an important predictor. Having two first-degree relatives with this disease raises risk by a factor of 18; three or more relatives with the disease equates to a 57-fold increase in risk.[4] BRCA mutation carriers have increased lifetime risk that is still quite small: 2 percent with a BRCA1 mutation and 3 to 5 percent with a BRCA2 mutation.[5] Inherited mutations are linked to about 10 percent of pancreatic cancers, even when there's no family history of the disease. If pancreatic cancer runs in your family, consult with a genetics specialist to determine your risk and to develop a plan for risk management.

> **PREVIVOR OR SURVIVOR?**
>
> If you've ever been diagnosed with cancer, you're a *survivor*. You're a *previvor* if you have a family history of disease, an inherited mutation, or other factor that predisposes you to developing cancer and you've never been diagnosed.

Melanoma

People with mutations in BRCA2 have a slightly increased risk for melanoma, an aggressive and deadly form of cancer that affects the skin and eyes. Excessive exposure to sunlight is a risk factor for both cancers, especially if you have naturally blonde or red hair, fair skin, and blue or green eyes. Melanoma of the eye often presents no symptoms, especially in its early stages. It may cause blurred vision in one eye, floaters (small spots that move around in your field of vision), a spot or a change of color on the iris, pain in the eye, or loss of peripheral vision. The lifetime risk for BRCA2-related melanoma is about 5 percent.[6]

Prostate Cancer

Men with BRCA mutations have increased risk for prostate cancer (discussed in chapter 17).

WHAT TO REMEMBER ABOUT BREAST AND OVARIAN CANCER

- Breast cancer may develop with no noticeable symptoms.
- Many women who develop ovarian cancer do have symptoms.
- Breast cancer is often discovered in its early, most treatable stages. Ovarian cancer is not.
- Most cancers aren't caused by an inherited mutation.

LEARN MORE ABOUT BREAST AND OVARIAN CANCER

The American Cancer Society (www.cancer.org) offers information and support related to prevention, treatment, and research involving all types of cancers.

Susan G. Komen for the Cure (www.cancer.org) and www.breastcancer .org provide up-to-date information about breast cancer.

The National Ovarian Cancer Coalition (www.ovarian.org) and the Ovarian Cancer National Alliance (www.ovariancancer.org) provide support and information related to ovarian cancer.

Chapter 2   A Peek Inside

Your Genes at Work

FEW AREAS OF SCIENCE HAVE CHANGED THE WORLD of medicine more in the past fifty years than genetics, the study of hereditary characteristics and variations passed from parent to child. With capabilities previously unimagined, scientists use genetic processes to trace ancestry, examine fossils, and make foods more disease resistant. Because most diseases, including breast and ovarian cancers, are caused at least in part by changes in the genes, this science is the key to understanding the origins of disease. Blood tests can now detect genetic changes that can cause diseases, from cystic fibrosis in a newborn to breast and ovarian cancer in an adult. Knowing about these genetic disorders can be life changing, because it provides opportunities to reduce the likelihood of developing the disease or to manage it early on. These discoveries are amazing, yet they only scratch the genetic surface. The more scientists understand what causes genetic abnormalities that lead to cancer, the closer we move toward better prevention, detection, treatment, and cure.

The Evolution of Genetic Discovery: From Peas to BRCA

In 1866, Austrian monk Gregor Mendel, considered the father of genetics, made a stunning declaration based on his experiments cross-breeding pea plants: that "factors" (now called genes) determine traits that are passed unchanged to descendants, and for each trait, individuals inherit one gene from each parent. Science ultimately proved Mendel correct and his conclusions became the tenets of modern genetics. Genes pass from parent to child, along with abnormalities within the genes that raise a person's risk for disease.

In 1990, genetics researcher Dr. Mary-Claire King demonstrated that a single inherited gene mutation causes breast and ovarian cancer among multiple members in some families. The link between the two cancers had been suspected since the late 1800s; now researchers had a clue for further exploration. Her proof that breast cancers could be inherited paved the way for subsequent research. King documented the general location of the "breast cancer" gene. A frenzy of subsquent research followed, and in 1994, scientists documented the precise location of BRCA1, the first breast cancer gene, on chromosome 17. BRCA2 was identified on chromosome 13 the following year. Now researchers knew exactly where to find these two genes, and a blood test was developed to screen individuals for cancer-causing BRCA mutations.

In the same year Dr. King announced her discovery, the Human Genome Project was launched to identify the entire set of human genes. By 2003, researchers had successfully labeled all 20,000 or so genes and created a genetic road map showing where each could be found. The massive effort was akin to translating every book ever written into a universal language: the genetic code that enables researchers to study what each gene does and how abnormalities cause disease. Even though it will be several years before we have all the answers, the increasing pace of genetic discoveries is rapidly advancing our knowledge of disease. Because genes appear in exactly the same order in all of us, knowing the location of a particular disease-causing gene is a huge medical leap forward. We now know where to find more than four thousand genes related to diseases, including many cancers.

Discovering BRCA1/2 was an important step in identifying high-risk individuals and finding ways to reduce their breast and ovarian cancer risk. As we learn more about BRCA mutations, our arsenal of risk management tools and cancer treatments grows. We still have much to learn about hereditary cancer. We don't know why some people with mutations get breast cancer and others develop ovarian cancer, or why some never have either disease. We can't predict when cancer will develop or how individuals will respond to treatment. And there may be as-yet undiscovered gene mutations that also raise cancer risk. Future genetic discoveries will provide those answers, ultimately leading to methods that will eradicate these diseases.

Your Genetic ABCs . . . and a D

Genetics is a complex science with its own unique language. Understanding the basics helps to clarify how changes in BRCA genes can lead to increased cancer risk.

A is for All of Us

Geraniums, worms, poodles, and humans—all living organisms have the same fundamental microscopic cells that keep us operating. Humans have trillions of cells, each with the same basic structure, yet programmed for very specific tasks like breathing, converting food into energy, and sending messages to and from the brain. You have an almost unimaginable assortment of cells, and most of them contain a complete set of your genetic material sufficient to create an exact copy of you.

B is for the Basics

Within each of our cells (except red blood cells) is a genetic control center called the nucleus. Every nucleus has twenty-three pairs of chromosomes: one of each pair comes from your mother; the other is from your father. Chromosomes are composed of snippets of genetic material that store and transmit the operating instructions that keep our bodies functioning. Genes also come in pairs (except those in egg and sperm cells), one from each parent. Genes work together to determine specific human characteristics, such as height or hair color, that pass from one generation to the next. When someone says, "It's in your genes," they're referring to a characteristic that's very much like one of your parent's. They might mean the curly hair both you and your mother have or the artistic ability you share with your father. Some genetic characteristics, such as eye color or the shape of your hairline, don't affect your health or well-being. Others may cause traits like color blindness or make you more likely to develop diseases such as diabetes or breast cancer.

C is for Cells

We all begin life as a single cell that grows and divides. Those two cells then divide and become four, and so on and so on, until our bodies are formed. This replicating life cycle is normally carried out in an orderly process controlled by genes: some tell cells when to divide, and others put the brakes on cell growth.

D is for DNA

You've probably heard of DNA, which stands for *deoxyribonucleic acid*, the unique genetic material used to link suspects to crime scenes, prove someone's paternity, or screen for certain mutations that lead to disease. All humans share about 99.9 percent of our DNA. Yet, except for identical twins, no two people are exactly alike. That's because our individual one-tenth of a percent variation determines our inherited

A genetic portrait of your DNA

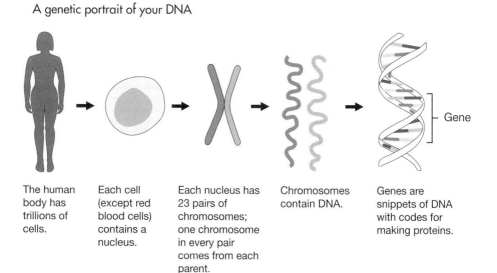

| The human body has trillions of cells. | Each cell (except red blood cells) contains a nucleus. | Each nucleus has 23 pairs of chromosomes; one chromosome in every pair comes from each parent. | Chromosomes contain DNA. | Genes are snippets of DNA with codes for making proteins. |

traits, like eye color and hair texture. Although you and your sister have genes that determine eye color, your variation of those genes may have resulted in your eyes being brown, while your sister's unique genetic variation gave her hazel eyes.

Genes perform an incredibly important job. These tightly coiled sections of thin DNA fibers issue instructions for making the thousands of proteins that build and support the body's elaborate operations—move muscles, digest food, repair cell damage. We hear a lot these days about genes, but proteins—often referred to as the body's building blocks—are the chemicals of life, and every cellular function depends on them. Genes instruct cells which proteins to make based on the type of cell and its needs. Some, like BRCA genes, tell our bodies how to repair damage from sun exposure, chemicals, and other influences. Others maintain just the right number of cells—enough to keep the body healthy, but not too many to encourage tumor growth. Cells, chromosomes, DNA, genes, proteins—mix these elements together uniquely and the result is: you.

Mutations: Spelling Errors in Your DNA Cookbook

Think of DNA as your body's cookbook, where your genes are recipes for proteins made by your body. DNA recipes are written in a sort of biological shorthand using various combinations of a four-letter alphabet, each representing a different chemical base: A (adenine), C (cytosine), G (guanine), and T (thymine). By combining different variations of these four "letters" into three-letter "words," DNA issues instructions for all the proteins our bodies need. The unique order of these letters spells out recipes for making everything from

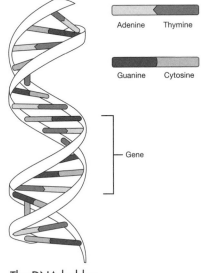

The DNA ladder

Table 3. Genetic spelling errors

Intended recipe	Mutation (spelling error)	Result
Add one big egg	Delete one letter (recipe begins in the wrong place and words shift)	Ddo neb ige gg
	Insert one letter (recipe shifts)	Add don ebi geg g
	Substitute letters	Add one bug egg
	Rearrangements	Egg add one big

hormones to heart valves. Under the microscope, DNA molecules look like the rungs of a ladder made up of A-T and C-G pairs.

If you use a cake recipe that includes a typo, your dessert might not turn out the way it should. The same thing happens when genetic changes called mutations create "spelling errors" that garble a DNA recipe for a specific protein. Different types of spelling errors may occur (see table 3).

Some spelling errors completely change the recipe and make it unreadable. Insertions and deletions cause words to shift, resulting in nonsense. Substitution errors can create sentences made up of real words that have different meanings: adding a "bug" egg instead of a "big" egg ruins the recipe. Sometimes, even though all the right letters are there, they end up in the wrong place, or words become scrambled and create meaningless sentences, creating mutations called *rearrangements*.

Most mutations aren't harmful. Some play an important evolutionary role, like changing an animal's appearance or behavior in ways that better adapt it to its surroundings. In some cases, the end result of mutations is disease. Sickle cell anemia, for instance, occurs when a mutation disrupts the instructions for hemoglobin, a protein made by red blood cells to move oxygen through the bloodstream. Mutations can also develop naturally as we grow older, as the wear and tear of living takes its toll on our recuperative abilities, and our genetic repair mechanisms don't work as effectively as they used to. Cells often develop mutations when they divide, and other mutations occur as a result of environmental and lifestyle influences, such as chemical exposure, radiation, smoking, and alcohol. The body frequently repairs genetic damage before the mutation is copied to new cells. Damage that cannot be repaired creates a bit of a vicious cycle: when a damaged cell divides, it passes all its DNA code, including any unrepaired mutations, on to the next generation of new cells. That error is then copied every time the new cell duplicates itself. If an error occurs in the egg or sperm, it may pass from parent to child in successive generations.

How Mutations Lead to Cancer

Not all cells divide—brain and heart cells don't. Those that do are more likely to develop mutations. Experts believe that cancer develops when both copies of certain genes in one cell are damaged and can't be repaired. Healthy cells usually repair DNA damage. Having two copies of each damage-repairing gene acts as a backup repair system: if one gene can't repair damage, the other can. That's why being born with a single BRCA mutation doesn't guarantee you'll develop breast or ovarian cancer, because your remaining BRCA gene can repair damage. If you develop a single error in that remaining protective BRCA gene, the damage control process is deactivated, and the gene no longer makes proteins to repair damage within the cells. When that first cell divides, it creates more damaged, unregulated copies of

How cell mutations evolve into cancer

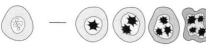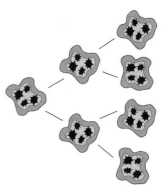

Normal cell   Cell mutations   Uncontrolled growth

itself. These cells are then free to run amok, growing and dividing beyond their normal lifespan and forming a tumor. On average, a breast tumor develops over six to eight years before it's large enough to be found by a mammogram, and about ten years before it can be felt. The process may occur sooner in people with hereditary mutations because the first step in cancer development—disabling one copy of the protective gene—has already occurred.

GENE THERAPY: A GLIMPSE INTO THE FUTURE

When cars malfunction or limbs break, we fix them. Can we do the same with rogue genes? Scientists are studying ways to repair faulty genes or override their cancer-causing ways. Someday, mutated BRCA genes might be fixed or swapped for healthy replacements.

EXPERT VIEW: Gene Variations and Breast Cancer Risk

BY KENNETH OFFIT, M.D., M.P.H.

Two categories of genes are associated with increased breast cancer risk. The first are genes in which mutations are quite rare, including BRCA1 and BRCA2, TP53, PTEN, STK11, and others, which are associated with greatly increased risk. A subset of this group includes ATM, CHEK2, BRIP1, PALB2, and other genes with rare mutations that are linked to much higher risks than those in the general population yet lower than with BRCA.

The second group includes a number of *single-nucleotide polymorphisms* (SNPs), genetic variations that only slightly increase breast cancer risk.

(continued)

Although SNPs occur in 10 to 30 percent or more of the population, the risk for breast cancer they cause is small: a 1.1- to 1.3-fold increased risk for individual SNPs compared to the 20- to 50-fold increased risk for breast cancer from BRCA mutations. Adding these new genetic variants to traditional risk models such as the Gail Model (see chapter 3) provides little new information that is clinically useful.

For now, SNPs are still poorly understood by scientists and best used in research. Although commercial laboratories market breast cancer SNP tests to the public, the American Society of Clinical Oncology and other professional groups caution about the potential harms of using unproven tests to determine risk. Several research groups are exploring whether SNPs can explain multiple cases of breast cancer in families who have no mutations in known breast cancer genes.

BRCA1 and BRCA2 testing continues to represent only the tip of the iceberg in pinpointing the link between genes and cancer risk, yet it remains the most reliable means to assess hereditary risk. In the future, we can expect more extensive evaluation of an individual's complete genetic information and a better understanding of how variations among genes can predispose us to disease. This will provide people with estimates of their risk for cancer and other diseases, as well as their sensitivities to certain environmental exposures and to drugs that may be prescribed to prevent breast and other cancers.

What's So Special about BRCA?

Hereditary breast and ovarian cancer doesn't develop because we have BRCA genes; everyone has them. It's mutations in these genes that cause disease. BRCA1 and BRCA2 are important because they're *tumor-suppressor* genes—their normal role is to stop cancer from developing by helping cells repair DNA damage. Most hereditary breast and ovarian cancers are caused by mutations in these genes. Mutations in other tumor-suppressor genes may also cause cancer.

Although BRCA mutations are found in all races and ethnicities, they're most prevalent in people of Ashkenazi Jewish descent. One in 40 will test positive, compared to 1 in 350 to 500 in the general population.[1] At some point far back in history, Ashkenazi ancestors developed DNA defects in some of their genes, including in BRCA1 and BRCA2. These *founder* mutations have been passed from generation to generation with greater frequency than in other populations because the Ashkenazi have lived in relative isolation, maintaining their common gene pool. About 40 percent of Jewish women with ovarian cancer and 20 percent who have premenopausal breast cancer have a BRCA mutation—a much higher rate than non-Jewish populations. Some Hispanic people (mostly those of Mexican heritage) carry the same mutation commonly found in Ashkenazi Jews, possibly due to a shared Spanish ancestry.[2] BRCA mutations also occur more often among Icelanders, Norwegians, Dutch, French Canadians, and other ethnic groups with relatively small numbers of ancestors.

You're more likely to have a BRCA mutation if your family has any of the following features:

- Ashkenazi Jewish heritage
- Any family member with
    - ovarian, fallopian tube, or primary peritoneal cancer at any age
    - breast cancer at age 50 or younger
    - breast cancer in both breasts at any age
    - both breast and ovarian cancer
    - male breast cancer
- More than one relative on the same side of the family with
    - breast cancer
    - ovarian, fallopian tube, or primary peritoneal cancer
    - prostate cancer
    - pancreatic cancer

WHAT TO REMEMBER ABOUT GENETICS

- All humans have exactly the same number of genes.
- Genetic mutations can be acquired or inherited.
- Mutations can interfere with a gene's ability to repair cellular damage.
- Cancer occurs when cells grow uncontrollably.

LEARN MORE ABOUT GENETICS

Genetics Home Reference (ghr.nlm.nih.gov) is a comprehensive guide for understanding genetics, including an A-to-Z guide to genetic conditions.

A Revolution in Progress: Human Genetics and Medical Research (history.nih.gov/exhibits/genetics/index.htm) is an illustrated introduction to the genetic influence on disease.

Breakthrough: The Race to Find the Breast Cancer Gene, by Kevin Davies and Michael White, describes the historic efforts to identify the BRCA1 gene.

Chapter 3 Defining Risk

DO YOU WORRY about getting malaria? Probably not if you live in the United States, where our risk of that disease is slim. But like many women, you may fear your risk of cancer, especially when you hear that 1 in 8 women will develop breast cancer. This means that, based on current rates of breast cancer in the entire U.S. population of women, 1 of 8 women born now will develop the disease by age 85. That sounds like a lot, but it also means that 7 of 8 women won't be diagnosed. Ovarian cancer occurs less often; the average woman has just a 1 in 70 chance in her lifetime.

The 1 in 8 and 1 in 70 estimates represent the average woman's risk for breast and ovarian cancer, yet these are broad statistics that don't define what you need to know to address your own risk: what is it now and how will it change as you grow older? If you're 20 years old now with an average risk for breast cancer, you have a 1 in 8 chance of being diagnosed in your lifetime. Your current risk isn't 1 in 8. It's much lower and gradually increases as you age (most risk occurs after

U.S. lifetime breast and ovarian cancer rates

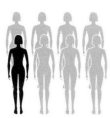

Breast cancer: 1 in 8

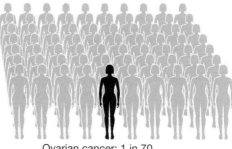

Ovarian cancer: 1 in 70

age 50). Until we know all the causes of cancer, we can't be sure about an individual's exact risk. In the meantime, scientists use population-based figures to describe the frequency of a disease, to help public health officials develop screening guidelines, and to determine cancer trends.

Making Sense of Statistics

Breast cancer is one of the most studied diseases in the world, yet most women don't know much about their own risk. Even fewer understand their odds of developing ovarian cancer. The concept of cancer risk can be confusing—just hearing *risk* is chilling—and because it's often expressed in different ways, understanding how it applies to you can be difficult.

CALCULATING THE 1 IN 8 STATISTIC

The current 1 in 8 statistic is calculated by the National Cancer Institute based on breast cancer rates in the United States between 2001 and 2003, when 12.5 percent of women were diagnosed. That statistic will change as breast cancer rates increase or decrease.

Certain factors raise your likelihood of disease: having high blood pressure increases your chance of developing heart disease, obesity boosts the odds of diabetes, and inheriting a BRCA mutation significantly raises your probability for breast and ovarian cancer. There are many reasons why your chance of developing cancer differs from someone else's, and therein lies the complexity, if not the impossibility, of pinpointing a person's exact risk. Your own risk of breast cancer isn't 1 in 8 because you're not average. It's a moving target that changes throughout your lifetime, depending on your family history, age, race and ethnicity, lifestyle, and other factors that shift your odds of developing cancer higher or lower than the population average. Although risk assessment is never an exact science, it's becoming more precise as researchers continue to learn about factors that influence cancer. Fortunately, genetics experts can assess different aspects of your personal medical history and family history to help you better predict and understand your risk. Confronting that risk may be frightening, but it's critical to do so, especially if you're genetically predisposed to one or more cancers, because if your risk is high, you have options for managing it.

EXPERT VIEW: Risk Assessment Using the Gail Model

BY VICTORIA SEEWALDT, M.D.

Experts use several tools, including the popular Gail Model, to estimate a woman's breast cancer risk. This model considers a woman's most common risk factors compared to women in the general population, based on her age; her age at first childbirth and menstrual period; whether her mother, sister, or daughter had breast cancer; and the number of breast biopsies she's had. It isn't the best way to determine hereditary breast cancer risk for several reasons:

- The model takes into account only first-degree female relatives, ignoring all other relatives including paternal history.
- It doesn't consider other cancers that can increase risk, such as ovarian cancer in a female relative or male breast cancer.
- It doesn't take into account the age when breast cancer occurs.
- It underestimates breast cancer risk in women of color.

MY STORY: The Gail Model Didn't Work for Me

My mother was diagnosed at age 31 and died four years later. My grandmother and great-grandmother also had breast cancer, and I wondered if there was a hereditary link. I asked my primary care physician about genetic testing, reminding him that my mother had been diagnosed at my age. He told me his nurse had just received a risk tool called the Gail Model that could assess my risk. Based on my answers to just seven questions, she determined I wasn't at high risk. I was relieved, but I couldn't stop thinking about one of the questions she had asked repeatedly: "How many of your sisters or your mother's sisters developed breast cancer?" My answer had been zero, because neither of us had any sisters. Would a different answer affect my risk assessment? I realized the test didn't apply to me because I

(continued)

had few female relatives. I needed someone more qualified, and that led
me to genetic counseling and then genetic testing, which showed I have a
BRCA1 mutation and my risk is actually quite high.   —JORDAN

Getting Personal: Factors That Modify Your Risk

Risk is the probability of something occurring at a certain time. When you drive to work each day, you take the chance of getting stuck in traffic or being rear-ended. Climb a ladder and you risk falling off. We're all susceptible to the risk of developing certain cancers, even though our risk is not the same. Having one or more risk factors—including a BRCA mutation—doesn't guarantee you'll develop cancer. It means you're more likely to do so. Smoking, for example, increases the odds of developing lung cancer. Stop smoking, and you decrease that risk. Obesity is a contributing risk factor for some diseases; maintaining a healthy weight has the opposite effect. You can control numerous lifestyle factors to reduce your risk; others you cannot. The following factors affect breast and ovarian cancer risk in the general population and, in some cases, may also influence risk in women with BRCA mutations.

Breast and ovarian cancer risk factors you cannot control:

- Being female. All women are at risk for breast and ovarian cancer.
- Growing older. Your risk increases as you age, whether or not you have a BRCA mutation.
- Personal history of breast cancer. Surviving breast cancer increases your risk for another diagnosis whether or not you have a BRCA mutation. The risk is greater for women with mutations.
- Inheriting a genetic mutation. Having a BRCA mutation raises the risk for breast and ovarian cancer more than any other factor. Other inherited mutations may also raise cancer risk (discussed in chapter 4).
- A family history of breast or ovarian cancer. Having a family history of cancer influences risk, although it's difficult to predict how much. About 1 in 4 women with breast cancer has a relative who has also been diagnosed; most don't have a BRCA mutation. If your family has

multiple members with breast cancer, no history of ovarian cancer, and no known BRCA mutation, your estimated lifetime risk for breast cancer is 20 to 25 percent.[1] Your lifetime risk for ovarian cancer is 1.4 percent (the same as an average woman's).[2] Having relatives diagnosed with ovarian cancer raises your risk for a similar diagnosis, even when you have no known mutation. Within BRCA families, having more cancers among relatives appears to cause higher breast and ovarian cancer risk for women family members. No matter what your family history, a genetics expert can help explain your personal risk.

- Race and ethnicity. Certain populations are more likely to develop breast cancer. Compared to white women, African American women have lower rates of breast and ovarian cancer but are more likely to be diagnosed before age 40. Their breast tumors are often particularly aggressive or triple-negative cancers that don't respond to hormone-blocking therapy, and their breast cancer mortality rate is higher than any other group of U.S. women.[3] Hispanic women are also diagnosed less frequently than their white counterparts. When they develop breast cancer, their tumors are more likely to be advanced. Among Asian women, breast cancer occurs less frequently, but it's increasing at a faster rate.

- Very high radiation exposure. Receiving radiation to your chest as a child or young adult elevates your risk of developing breast cancer later in life.

- Age at first menstruation. Early menarche increases the risk for breast cancer in the general population and may have the same effect in women with BRCA mutations.

- Previous breast biopsies. Having any number of biopsies, especially if they showed certain precancerous breast changes, can indicate increased breast cancer risk.

- Breast density. Women with dense breast tissue have greater risk of developing breast cancer, LCIS, and other precancerous abnormalities.

- Infertility. Though research is limited and the connection is unclear, infertility has been linked to increased breast cancer risk in BRCA carriers and to breast and ovarian cancer risk in the general population.

Breast and ovarian cancer risk factors you can modify:

You can't totally eliminate your risk for cancer, but you can change your behavior to reduce your risk. The following factors affect breast and ovarian cancer risk to different degrees in the general population and, in some cases, also influence risk in BRCA carriers. In subsequent chapters, you'll read more about how you can modify these lifestyle factors to change your risk.

- Pregnancy. Being pregnant affects breast cancer risk in complex ways. For all women, a first pregnancy while young lowers risk—the younger you are, the more beneficial the effect. If you're a previvor, your risk may also be affected by your number of pregnancies and whether you have a mutation in BRCA1 or BRCA2.
- Oral contraceptives. Using oral contraceptives while young and continuing for more than five years may increase breast cancer risk in women with BRCA mutations (research is limited). On the other hand, oral contraceptives lower the chance for ovarian cancer in all women.
- Tubal ligation. In the general population, tying a woman's tubes may lower her risk for ovarian cancer, although not as much as oral contraceptives do. Whether this is true for high-risk women is unknown.
- Hormone replacement therapy. Women of average breast cancer risk who take combined estrogen and progesterone hormone replacement after natural menopause have increased risk for breast and ovarian cancer. Hormones may be safer for previvors who pre-emptively remove their breasts and ovaries than for women in the general population, who have undergone natural menopause.
- Alcohol consumption. Having one or more drinks a day elevates the chance of breast cancer in women of average risk. Researchers aren't sure whether women with BRCA mutations are affected in the same way.
- Exercise and obesity. Evidence suggests that physical activity and maintaining an ideal body weight (avoiding obesity) lower the odds of developing breast cancer in women of average or high risk.
- Breast reduction. Some preliminary (and not widely validated) research indicates that breast cancer risk is reduced after breast reduction surgery.

- Removing both breasts and ovaries. These aggressive preventive actions reduce your risk.

It's a Numbers Game

Calculating someone's precise risk for BRCA-related breast and ovarian cancer is difficult. It's a field that is still evolving, and we simply don't know everything about it, including other genes or factors that might also influence risk. BRCA risk estimates are calculated from studies of large multicancer families, and it's unclear how much risk is due to genetic mutations or environmental influences shared by family members. In the absence of finite predictions, genetics experts use a range of numbers to describe a person's odds of developing cancer; even this range of risk varies. Experts may not agree on the exact numbers, but they do agree that inheriting a BRCA mutation means higher-than-average risk that warrants increased surveillance or risk-reducing strategies.

Absolute and Relative Risk

It's important to understand two distinctly different types of risk. *Absolute risk* is the chance of getting cancer over a certain period. The 1 in 8 breast cancer statistic, for example, expresses an average woman's lifetime risk if she lives to age 85. Absolute risk is never less than 0 or more than 100 percent. *Relative risk* is

YOUR BELIEFS AND CULTURE MAY AFFECT HOW YOU CONFRONT YOUR RISK

We all have different ideas about medicine and cancer risk that are often shaped by how we were raised, our family beliefs, and our observations of others who have been diagnosed. Concerns about modesty may prevent you from learning more about cancers of your breasts and ovaries or even speaking about these issues. Social and economic influences may keep you from performing self-exams, having routine mammograms, or changing lifestyle behaviors that affect your risk. Some cultures consider illness to be a *fait accompli*; it's accepted as a destiny we can't control, so why worry about it or try to prevent it? Perhaps you're mistrustful or disillusioned because you can't find a physician who speaks your preferred language. You may feel stigmatized by a cancer diagnosis and delay recommended treatment. Culture and shared values connect us to family and community, which provide our support system, but sometimes it's wise to take a step back and assess if our beliefs help or hinder how we approach important health issues.

Lifetime breast and ovarian cancer risk as a percentage

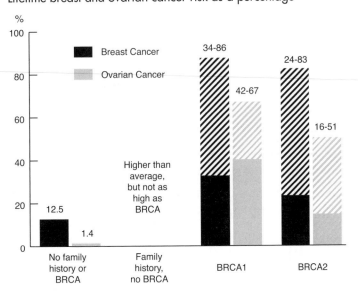

Source: Data for BRCA1 and BRCA2 taken from Chen S and Parmigiani G, "Meta-Analysis of BRCA1 and BRCA2 Penetrance," *Journal of Clinical Oncology* 25, no. 11 (2007): 1329–33.

a percentage of increase or decrease calculated by comparing people who have a particular risk factor with people who don't; in other words, a smoker compared to a nonsmoker. Consider an average woman whose lifetime risk for breast cancer is 12.5 percent. Something that inflates her relative risk by 10 percent raises her absolute risk to 13.75 percent (12.5 + 1.25). If a woman with a BRCA2 mutation takes medication that lowers her ovarian cancer risk by 50 percent, her relative risk is then half of what it was compared to a woman with the mutation who doesn't take the medication.

MY STORY: I Assumed My Risk Was 100 Percent

Because I had atypical ductal hyperplasia (ADH), and my mother and both grandmothers had breast cancer, my breast surgeon said I had a very high risk of getting it too. I always thought I would somehow escape the breast cancer that ran in my family. Once I had ADH, I felt 100 percent certain

I would follow in my mother's and grandmothers' footsteps, so I had my breasts removed. I found out later that I don't have a mutation.   —KRIS

Knowing your lifetime risk for cancer has limited value when you're considering ways to manage your current risk. Addressing your risk over a specific timeframe is particularly important if you have a BRCA mutation, because you're more likely to be diagnosed with breast cancer before age 50. Understanding your incremental risk is also important when considering treatment options. A woman with sporadic breast cancer may choose breast-conserving surgery, knowing her risk for another tumor in ten years is just 10 percent. A woman with BRCA-related breast cancer might prefer mastectomy instead, because her risk of a second cancer over the same period is 30 percent.

EXPERT VIEW: Decade-by-Decade Risks

BY TIMOTHY R. REBBECK, PH.D.

The numbers in table 4 (see page 34) were derived from Johns Hopkins University researchers who combined nine studies that estimate cancer risks in BRCA mutation carriers. Combining studies to obtain composite risk estimates is a good way to provide more representative numbers when trying to understand risk variations across many small populations, as we see in BRCA carriers. Each study reported different risk results. These differences can be explained by how the studies were analyzed, which families and individuals were included, the total number of individuals who were included, and other factors. Table 4 supplies our best estimate of decade-by-decade and lifetime risk for BRCA1 and BRCA2 mutation carriers based on the aggregate of all nine studies. As we study more people with BRCA mutations, we gain a better idea of risk. It is important to remember that risk varies considerably between women: the estimates in table 4 represent an average risk across all populations. An individual's risk may be quite different from the average.

(continued)

Table 4. Average probability of developing breast or ovarian cancer

	Breast cancer risk with BRCA1 mutation (%)	Breast cancer risk with BRCA2 mutation (%)	Ovarian cancer risk with BRCA1 mutation (%)	Ovarian cancer risk with BRCA2 mutation (%)
By age 30	< 1	1	almost none	almost none
By age 40	2	10	4	2
By age 50	14	22	14	2
By age 60	32	36	28	10
By age 70	47	49	40	18
By age 80	57	49	40	18
Lifetime	64	56	55	31

Source: Chen S and Parmigiani G, "Meta-Analysis of BRCA1 and BRCA2 Penetrance," Journal of Clinical Oncology 25, no. 11 (2007): 1329–33.

THE FORCE (FACING OUR RISK OF CANCER EMPOWERED) PERSPECTIVE: PUTTING MEDIA REPORTS INTO CONTEXT

Media stories about behaviors, foods, or other factors that raise or reduce cancer risk can be misleading if not put into proper context. Hearing that 1 in 10 women is obese by age 40 doesn't necessarily apply to you because your personal risk for obesity is different, depending on factors you can control: exercising regularly and eating balanced meals in proper proportions. Similarly, hearing that "exercise reduces breast cancer risk by 50 percent" doesn't necessarily mean your risk is half that of your couch-potato neighbor if you jog every day. The next time you hear one of these encouraging or scary reports, consider it with caution and talk to your doctor about how it may or may not affect you.

WHAT TO REMEMBER ABOUT RISK

- BRCA risk is a best guess based on current research.
- Risk is a moving target that changes throughout your lifetime.

- You can control certain risk factors; others you cannot.
- Your genes don't necessarily define your destiny. No matter what your risk, you can take steps to manage it.

LEARN MORE ABOUT RISK

The National Cancer Institute has an online Breast Cancer Risk Assessment Tool (www.cancer.gov/bcrisktool).

In the Family (inthefamily.kartemquin.com) is an award-winning documentary that follows previvor Joanna Rudnick and several families affected by hereditary breast and ovarian cancer.

Assess Your True Risk of Breast Cancer, by Patricia Kelley, Ph.D., is a comprehensive guide to cancer risk.

Reduce Your Cancer Risk: Twelve Steps to a Healthier Life, by Barbara Boughton and Mike Stefanek, Ph.D., explains risk-reducing strategies.

Chapter 4 **Hereditary Cancer**

What's Swimming
in Your Gene Pool?

MUCH OF YOUR APPEARANCE results from traits you inherit from your parents. You can thank them for your cute dimples, stubby fingers, or widow's peak. These inherited characteristics are written into your DNA. You can pass them—and genetic mutations—on to your sons and daughters.

Mutations from Mom or Dad

All of us in the human race get half our genetic material from each parent. So it's equally possible to inherit a BRCA mutation from Mom or Dad. In fact, if we could identify every person with a BRCA mutation, we would find about half received their mutation from their father and half from their mother. If either of your parents has a BRCA mutation, you and each of your siblings have a 50 percent chance of inheriting it. Likewise, each of your children has the same 50 percent chance of inheriting your mutation and high cancer risk. Generally, children who don't inherit your mutation have average cancer risk.

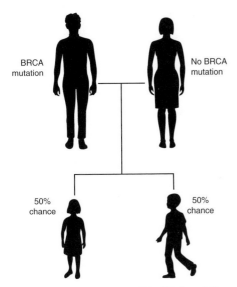

BRCA mutation

No BRCA mutation

50% chance

50% chance

Each child has a 50% chance of inheriting the mutation.

Probability of inheriting a mutation from one parent

Inheriting Multiple BRCA Mutations

While uncommon, it's possible to inherit mutations in both BRCA1 and BRCA2, especially if you're of Ashkenazi Jewish ethnicity. People with double mutations are believed to have risk for breast, ovarian, and fallopian cancer that is similar to individuals with BRCA1 mutations. Risk for melanoma, pancreatic cancer, prostate cancer, and male breast cancer is thought to be equivalent to someone with a BRCA2 mutation. If you have mutations in both BRCA genes, or you and your spouse each have a mutation, your risk of passing one or both mutations to your children is 75 percent. Embryos can grow with a double mutation in the BRCA2 gene, but they must have at least one working copy of BRCA1 to survive. Children who inherit a mutation in both copies of BRCA2—one mutation from each parent—develop Fanconi anemia (FA), a rare and serious childhood disorder characterized by bone marrow that doesn't produce enough blood cells. Several other genes are also linked with FA. Some children with this disorder have physical abnormalities such as altered skin pigment, deformed thumbs, a very small head size, or stunted growth. Other abnormalities in the heart, kidney, genitalia, or hearing may also develop. Blood abnormalities usually develop before age 12 and may include fatigue and paleness, bleeding or bruising, or susceptibility to infections from a low level of white blood cells.

Hidden Risk in the Family Tree

Sometimes it's difficult to determine whether a mutation runs in a family. Lifestyle choices, a small family size, having few female relatives, or having relatives who died early from other causes may obscure familial cancers. In some cases, family history may not be available. Many Ashkenazi Jewish families, for example, cannot trace their family history beyond the Holocaust. If you were adopted and don't know your family history, or your female relatives died before age 50 of unknown causes, a genetic counselor can help determine the likelihood that you inherited a mutation based on the information available.

Because either parent can pass a mutation to their children, ignoring Dad's side of the family can hide potential risk. Far fewer men than women with BRCA mutations develop cancer, potentially making indications of a mutation less obvious. Knowing the source of a mutation in your family can determine whether relatives on that side of the family may have the same mutation and associated high risk. A genetics expert can use your family history to try to determine whether a mutation came from your mother or father.

MY STORY: My Mutation Came from My Dad

Diagnosed with breast cancer, I thought I had no relevant family history. My father's first cousins had the disease; they were in their 60s and seemed like such distant relatives. I don't recall a single health form ever asking about my father's first cousin. After my diagnosis with breast cancer, I met with a genetic counselor who realized from my small family tree that my cancer likely came from my father's side. If he had more women on his side of the family, we may have seen more breast cancer. Sure enough, like my two cousins, I tested positive for a BRCA2 mutation.   —ELLYN

HBOC and Other Hereditary Cancer Syndromes

Hereditary cancer syndromes are caused by mutations that run in families and raise the risk of multiple cancers. BRCA mutations in a family cause hereditary breast and ovarian cancer (HBOC) syndrome, an inherited tendency for cancers of the breast, ovaries, fallopian tubes, pancreas, prostate, and skin. Several other cancer syndromes have been identified, each with a unique pattern of disease. Your family may have a hereditary cancer syndrome if multiple relatives have had certain types of cancers, including rare cancers; if the same cancer appears in more than one generation; or if cancers were diagnosed at a young age. One or two cases of the same types of cancer within a family—these days that includes many families—don't necessarily indicate a cancer

Table 5. Signs of HBOC within a family

Any blood relative with:	Ovarian or fallopian tube cancer at any age
	Breast cancer at age 50 or younger
	Breast cancer in both breasts at any age
	Both breast and ovarian cancer
	Male breast cancer
More than one relative on the same side of the family with:	Breast cancer
	Ovarian or fallopian tube cancer
	Prostate cancer
	Pancreatic cancer

syndrome. Any of the signs shown in table 5 may indicate that HBOC runs in the family.

Although HBOC is the most common cause of hereditary breast and ovarian cancer, inherited syndromes caused by mutations in other genes also increase the risk for these cancers.

Lynch Syndrome

Hereditary nonpolyposis colorectal cancer, also known as Lynch syndrome, increases risk for colon, uterine, and ovarian cancers. Women with Lynch syndrome have greater risk for ovarian cancer than other women, but less risk than someone who has a BRCA mutation. Caused by a mutation in one of several specific genes, Lynch syndrome is the most common hereditary cause of colon cancer, accounting for about 5 percent of all cases. If you have Lynch syndrome, you need regular screening at an early age—colonoscopy beginning between ages 20 and 25 is recommended—because you have a high risk for benign polyps that can develop into colon cancer if they're not removed during colonoscopy. Lynch syndrome may run in families in which a relative has been diagnosed with colorectal cancer more than once, when colorectal cancer or uterine cancer occurs in two successive generations in relatives age 50 or younger, or when three relatives have any of the cancers related to Lynch syndrome.

Cowden Syndrome

Cowden syndrome results from an inherited mutation in the PTEN tumor-suppressor gene. Even individuals who have no family history may develop the syndrome spontaneously. One in 200,000 people is estimated to have Cowden, with a risk of developing breast cancer as high as 50 percent.[1] Similar to individuals with BRCA mutations, diagnosis before age 50 may be more common. Only a small percentage of breast cancers are attributed to Cowden syndrome (it may be underdiagnosed). Having Cowden syndrome also ups the chance for other cancers, including thyroid (10 percent risk), endometrial (5 to 10 percent risk), and cancers of the kidney, colon, and skin (risk levels unknown). It's sometimes the underlying cause of otherwise unexplained cancers in families that test negative for a BRCA mutation.

Gene testing can identify this syndrome. It takes an experienced genetics expert to evaluate a family's unexplained cancers and determine if Cowden syndrome may be the culprit. Men and women with Cowden's have a higher-than-normal risk for both benign and cancerous growths including thyroid tumors; lesions of the skin, mouth, and lower digestive tract; and genital or uterine fibroids. Some studies have also linked PTEN mutations with melanoma and certain types of aggressive brain tumors. Other signs of this syndrome within a family are visible benign growths, such as lipomas (fatty lumps) or goiter (benign growth of the thyroid); polyps; hamartomas (benign masses); skin tags; fibrocystic breast changes; and intestinal polyps.

Li-Fraumeni Syndrome

Li-Fraumeni syndrome is caused by a rare inherited mutation in the P53 gene. This syndrome often causes childhood and adolescent cancers and carries a 50 to 80 percent risk of breast cancer between ages 15 and 44.[2] Individuals who have Li-Fraumeni often develop childhood cancers of the bone, soft tissue, adrenals, brain, stomach, and other organs.

Hereditary Diffuse Gastric Cancer Syndrome

Hereditary diffuse gastric cancer (HDGC) syndrome results from a mutation in the CDH1 gene. Little is known about HDGC. It can cause stomach cancers, often before age 40 (most gastric cancers in the general population are diagnosed after age 60). Women with an HDGC mutation have a 39 to 52 percent lifetime risk of developing lobular breast cancer.[3]

Peutz-Jeghers Syndrome

Peutz-Jeghers syndrome occurs from a mutation in the STK11 gene. Patients with this syndrome have elevated risk for breast and ovarian cancer, as well as cancer of the cervix, pancreas, and gastrointestinal tract. Children with Peutz-Jeghers often develop small dark freckles on the face, hands, feet, and anus that usually fade as they become teenagers. Thousands of polyps in the stomach and intestines are common in individuals with Peutz-Jeghers. It's a rare syndrome, and experts aren't sure how frequently it occurs.

Ataxia-Telangiectasia

Ataxia-telangiectasia (AT) is a rare disorder affecting only 1 in 100,000 births. It's believed to cause immune system cancers, including leukemia and lymphomas. Only individuals who inherit ATM gene mutations from both parents develop AT—but having a single mutation may predispose individuals to greater chance of developing breast cancer.

CDKN2A mutations

Mutations in the CDKN2A gene are also very rare. People who inherit this mutation have up to a 17 percent lifetime risk of pancreatic cancer and a 28 percent lifetime risk for melanoma.[4]

Plotting Your Genetic Pedigree

If your family has been affected by cancer, you've probably wondered about your own risk. A genetics expert can evaluate your family's pattern of disease to determine whether a mutation or hereditary cancer syndrome exists in your family, and whether you or a relative should consider genetic testing. First, you'll need to gather information to document your family's *pedigree*, or medical history. This document shows all your relatives, their relationship to you, and any diseases they've had. With this information, a genetic counselor can identify health patterns and determine your risk for inherited disease. Your pedigree can't predict your future health, but it can give you an insight your relatives never had: a peek into your future and the potential to change your fate by determining which diseases you're predisposed to develop.

Ideally, a genetics expert needs information from both sides of the family for three generations to determine whether a hereditary cancer pattern exists. So if possible, you'll need to collect information about your first-, second-, and third-degree biological relatives (see table 6).

Table 6. Gather information about three generations

First-degree relatives	Second-degree relatives	Third-degree relatives
siblings	half-siblings	cousins
children	uncles and aunts	great-grandparents
parents	grandparents	great-aunts and great-uncles
	grandchildren	
	nieces and nephews	